Homemade Skin Care

30 Recipes Made of Herbs and Essential Oils

Table of Contents

Introduction

I want to thank and congratulate you for downloading *"Essential Oils: Skin Care Recipes Made of Herbs and Essential Oils."* You need to take care of yourself inside and out, using my collection of skin care recipes will definitely help you to get your skin looking healthy once again. Feel good in knowing that you are using natural skin care homemade products to revitalize your skin. Before you know it you are going to feel and look ten years younger when you start to see the healthy and positive results from using my essential oil and herb based skin care recipes. Why pay a small fortune for products that have all kinds of artificial additives in them when instead you can use this skin care recipe collection that only used natural and healthy ingredients in the skin care recipes within these pages.

You are going to be so pleased with just how easy it really is to use your own homemade skin care products, that are not filled with harmful chemicals. I will teach you what essential oils are best to use on oily skin for example. I will also guide you on what essential oils you should use for full-body washing and facial care. You will also discover essential oils that work well together to help protect your skin.

Chapter 1. Using Essential Oils as Part of Your Skin Care Regimen

If you have never used essential oils as part of your skin care regimen, then I must tell you that you have been missing out on some of the most effective ingredients that can help your skin look and feel great. I am more than happy to share valuable information with you within the pages of this book about essential oils and how they 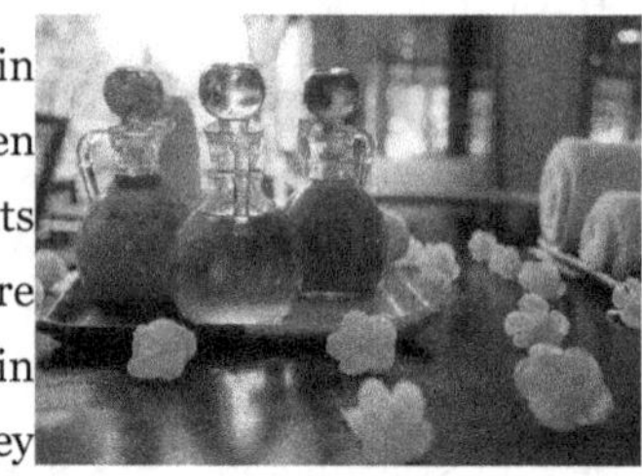 can benefit you. You will find that you will have healthy youthful looking skin in no time, with regular use of essential oils as part of your daily skin care regimen.

Why are they called "Essential Oils"?

The name itself actually is referring to a plant's "essence", rather than to how essential the oils are in skincare. The things that make plants what they are—the color, smell, and basic properties—are unique blends of organic molecules, aromatic compounds and phytonutrients. The essential oils are extracted from these plants and are distilled into concentrated liquids that contain within them the "essence" of the plants.

Essential oils smell wonderful, but this is not the most important feature of them. They are also very powerful, containing benefits that will improve your overall health, including your skin health. There is an essential oil for nearly any skin issue that you may have.

How to Use Essential Oils for Your Skin

There is a variety of different ways that you can use essential oil. They can be applied topically, which means that the application is absorbed through your skin. In this book I am targeting essential oils specifically for skin care. You may choose t include essential oils in DIY moisturizers or you can add them to formulas you already use in your daily skin care regimen.

Essential Oils Must be Diluted

Essential oils are very potent and must be diluted before you use them in your skin care. They are very powerful and concentrated and you only need a little to benefit from them. You will need to dilute your essential oils a lot using things such as carrier oils like coconut, hemp seed, jojoba and olive oil before you apply them to your skin. If you do not dilute essential oils they can cause irritation and sensitivity, and can even be toxic. You must only use them in the correct doses.

The Right Doses of Essential Oils

The total amount of the lotions or skin moisturizers you are using should be no more than two percent essential oils. If you have sensitive skin, you should probably only use one percent of essential oils in your skin care products. If for example your lotion is in a 12 ounce bottle then you can add 12 drops of essential oils to it. If you have sensitive skin then only add in 6 drops of essential oils. I know you are thinking that it does not sound like a lot, but keep in mind essential oils are very concentrated. So there is no sense using more than is needed.

If you are someone that suffers from acne you still do not have to add more essential oils, more is not better. Do not add more essential oils than is necessary as they are very potent and concentrated. You want to avoid irritating your skin further, do this by applying the essential oils as directed.

Exceptions to Dosing Rule

There is only a couple of essential oils that you can use full-strength or "neat", meaning undiluted. Tea tree oil and lavender oil can be used without diluting them. If you are using them in a moisturizer formula still use them at only 2%.

Most Effective Essential Oils for Acne & Oily Skin

You can gain many different kinds of benefits with the use of essential oils. They are very beneficial in treating acne and anti-aging. Both tea tree oil and lavender oil are popular to use in the treatment of oily skin. Some other essential oils that also work well with oily skin are neroli, clary, rosemary, geranium, rose, lemongrass, sage, sandalwood, chamomile, Calendula, helichrysum, myrrh and frankincense.

You can't Add them All to your Skin Care Products

After you become aware of the different benefits that each essential oil will offer, you might be tempted to add all of them into your skin care products. You simply cannot add all of them. Narrow your choices down based on the ones that suit your personal needs best. Choose essential oils that will address your skin conditions best.

If you want to use two of the best and most effective essential oils for oily skin I would suggest including frankincense and lavender oils. If you have not used them before only incorporate one oil at a time and see how it effects your skin. Take your time when you integrate a new essential oil into your daily skin care regimen. Take it even slower if you have sensitive skin. You want to use essential oils to help heal your skin not to irritate it. You do not want to make your skin even more sensitive by using too many new essential oils at once.

Do some research on the essential oils that you are interested in using as part of your skin care. Find out everything about them before you use them. You will want to choose essential oils that you will benefit the most from. For example if you use citrus oil it can create more photo-sensitivity in your skin. They should be used in skin care products only after you know they don't make your skin more photo-sensitive.

The Most Effective Kinds of Essential Oils

When you are going to choose your essential oils make sure you choose high quality brands. None of them will be cheap, but you do not want to spend less but get a poor quality of essential oil. These low-grade oils will not work like the high-quality ones will. Make sure when you purchase your essential oils that they are 100% pure. You do not want to use perfume oil, or fragrance oil.

You may also see that you can purchase some essential oils that have already been mixed with a carrier oil such as jojoba oil. You will be mixing your own 100% pure essential oils with a carrier oil of your choice. If of course you buy them with carrier oils already added then you do not need to add a carrier oil.

You will soon discover that 100% pure essential oils are not cheap. Prices can vary a lot, depending on what you want to use the oil for. It does take a lot of plant material to make just a small amount of essential oils. The higher quality essential oils are going to cost more. You may think that the prices seem rather high, since you are only buying small bottles of it. However, you need to keep in mind that they are highly concentrated and a little essential oil goes a long way. It is best to start with a couple of oils and then add on to your essential oil collection as you begin to learn what essential oils work best for you and your needs.

Chapter 2. Essential Oil Based Shower Gels, Bath Bombs & More

1. Tea Tree Essential Oil & Honey Mask

Honey is a product that is not used often enough, in my personal opinion. It is so wonderful for skin. When you use raw honey it will add antioxidants to your skin making it more youthful and vibrant Honey is a natural antibacterial, so it will help to moisturize your skin and unclog your pores and preventing acne. Tea tree 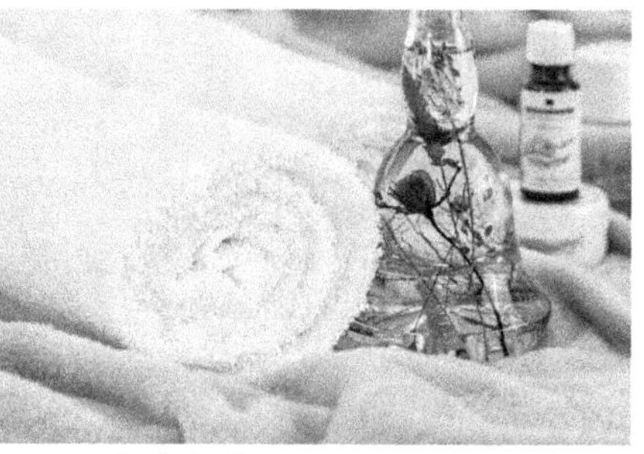 oil is a purifying oil, so it will certainly make a wonderful addition to your DIY mask.

Ingredients:

- 2 drops of essential tea tree oil

- 1 tablespoon of raw organic honey

Directions:

Place honey into small bowl. Mix in the two drops of tea tree oil. Apply this to your face and allow it to set for 30 minutes. Apply a light coat. Rinse your face with warm water.

2. *Essential Oil Shower Steamers*

Ingredients:

- 2 tablespoons of distilled water
- 10 drops of lavender essential oil
- 10 drops of frankincense essential oil
- 2 cups of baking soda
- 1 cup of citric acid

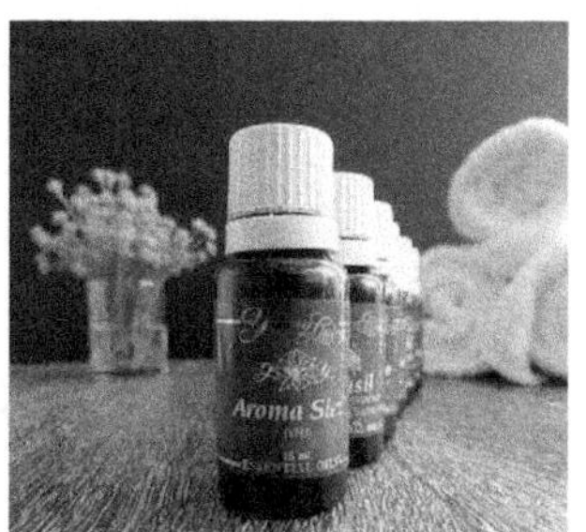

Directions:

Mix your citric acid and baking soda in a small bowl and set aside. Mix the essential oils and water together in a small sized dark glass bottle. Add in the oil mixture slowly into the baking soda mix. Stir well until it is well-blended. Pack the mixture into small balls of about 1-inch and then place them onto wax paper. Pack each ball tighter. Allow the balls to dry overnight. Keep them out of humidity and moisture.

3. Peppermint Essential Oil Bath Bombs

Ingredients:

- 1 cup of citric acid

- 10 drops of lemongrass essential oil

- 10 drops of peppermint essential oil

- 1 teaspoon of jojoba oil as a carrier

- 3 tablespoons of distilled water

- 1 cup of baking soda

- 1 bath bomb mold

Directions:

Mix the baking soda and citric acid in a small mixing bowl. Store essential oils and carrier oil in another bowl. Add the liquids to the soda mix and stir and blend well. Add into the mold. Mist the surface with water-filled spray bottle until it is a bit dense. Mix it until it has the consistency of wet sand. Do not add too much water or it will fall apart. Cover the mold using a paper towel, then turn it upside down onto a baking sheet. Tap the bottom of the mold gently and de-mold your bath bombs. Cover them with a paper towel and allow them to sit overnight to dry. Package your bath bombs in airtight bags or containers so they will keep their fizz.

4. *Lemon & Mint Essential Oil Sugar Scrub*

Ingredients:

- 5 drops of peppermint essential oil

- 5 drops of lemon essential oil

- 1 tablespoon of fresh lemon juice

- zest from half a lemon

- 1 and 1/4 cup of sugar, granulated

- 1/2 cup of coconut oil

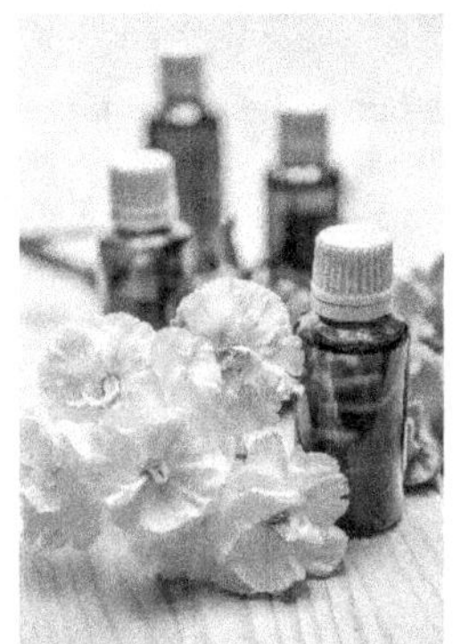

Directions:

Mix all of your ingredients in a mixing bowl. Make sure to blend them well. The zest and sugar will help to gently slough off dead skin cells, while the coconut oil will help to moisturize your skin. The lemon and peppermint essential oils will help to boost your mood!

5. *Essential Oil DIY Bath Detox*

Ingredients:

- 5 drops of lavender essential oil

- 5 drops of lemon essential oil

- 2 cups of Epsom salts

- 1 tablespoon of ginger, ground

Directions:

Mix your essential oils, Epsom salts, and ginger in a bowl. Mix well. Pour into a mason jar or similar jar and then secure the lid. Use this mix on those days when you want to soak in a relaxing essential oil bath.

6. *Oatmeal & Lavender Essential Oil DIY Body Wash*

Ingredients:

- 6 to 12 drops of lavender essential oil

- 1/4 cup of oatmeal

- 1/4 cup of liquid Castile soap

- 1 teaspoon of vitamin E oil

- 2 teaspoons of avocado or jojoba oil

- 3 cups of distilled water

- a foaming dispenser

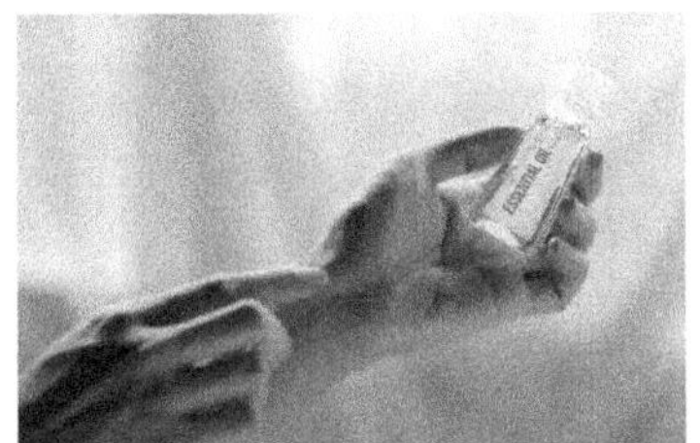

Directions:

Bring 3 cups of water to a low boil. Pour the water over the oatmeal in a small glass bowl. Allow it to sit for 2 hours. Strain the water to remove the oats. Discard the oats and set the water aside. Mix in the jojoba or avocado oil, vitamin E oil, essential oils, and Castile soap in a bowl. Whisk the mix. Pour the oil-soap mix into a foaming dispenser, only fill 10% of foam dispenser. Pour the oatmeal infused water into your dispenser until it is almost full. Twist the lid on to dispenser and you are ready to use it. This recipe will fill two average sized dispensers.

7. DIY Essential Oil Shower Gel

I thought it would be so cool to make a homemade shower gel, but I thought it would probably be too hard to do. However, I soon discovered that it was easy! You can make my shower gel in five minutes or less. It will give you lots of suds and will also moisturize your skin too. It is an all-natural recipe with no toxins in it. Once you become more familiar with essential oils and their scents you can begin to blend your favorite essential oils to make your own special shower gels. This recipe for shower gel smells wonderful!

Ingredients:

- 10 drops of ylang ylang essential oil

- 5 drops of blue spruce essential oil

- 1 teaspoon of vitamin E oil

- 1 teaspoon of jojoba oil—as a carrier oil

- 2/3 cup of Castile soap

- 2 tablespoons of raw organic honey

- 2 tablespoons of vegetable glycerin

Directions:

Whisk all of the ingredients and combine them well. Fill an eight ounce jar and secure onto it soap pump. You will just love the scent of this shower gel!

8. Essential Oil Acne Improvement Formula

Ingredients:

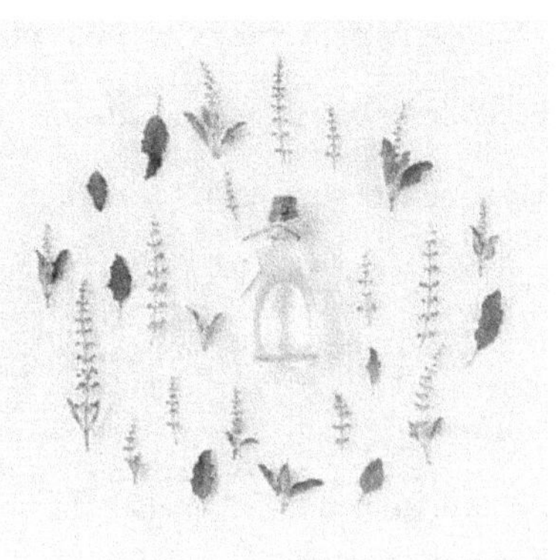

- 6 drops of tea tree essential oil

- 6 drops of lavender essential oil

- 6 drops of myrrh essential oil

- 6 drops of rosemary essential oil

- 3 tablespoons of hazelnut oil—as a carrier oil

- 1 tablespoon of jojoba oil—as carrier oil

Directions:

Mix all of your ingredients well in a bowl. Apply the mixture to blemishes with a clean finger or cotton pad. Myrrh is going to help with dissolving sebum (your skin's natural oil) for fewer acne breakouts. Jojoba oil is somewhat like sebum, so it can step into keep your skin nice and moist.

9. *DIY Essential Oil Facial Wash*

Ingredients:

- 16 drops of geranium essential oil
- 16 drops of bergamot essential oil
- 12 drops of tea tree essential oil
- 10 ounces of glycerin
- 4 ounces of Aloe Vera Gel

Directions:

Mix your ingredients well in a mixing bowl. Use a bit when you get up in the morning to wash your face, then rinse well.

10. *DIY Essential Oil Moisturizing Formula*

Ingredients:

- 5 drops of tea tree essential oil

- 10 drops of patchouli essential oil

- 5 drops of frankincense essential oil

- 5 drops of bergamot essential oil

- 5 drops of Ylang-Ylang essential oil

- 2 tablespoons of jojoba oil

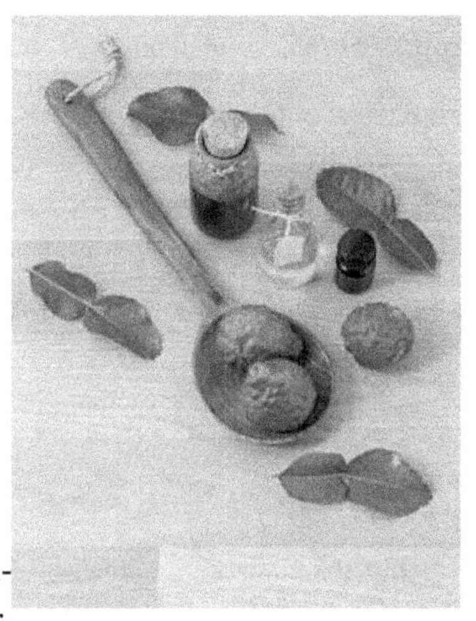

Directions:

Mix your ingredients together. Stir until well-blended. Use as needed as your moisturizer.

This is a basic formula, so once you have been using it for awhile you may choose to make some tweaks in it with the essential oils until you get a formula that suits your personal needs best. If you have sensitive skin you may choose to use lesser amounts of essential oils.

11. *Replenishing DIY Essential Oil Facial Serum*

Ingredients:

- 5 drops of Neroli essential oil

- 8 drops of geranium essential oil

- 8 drops of frankincense essential oil

- 8 drops of carrot seed essential oil

- 1 and 1/2 teaspoons of evening primrose oil

- 2 tablespoons of jojoba oil

Directions:

Blend all of your ingredients in a small glass bottle that has a dropper. Shake well before using. Add one or two drops to your throat and face.

12. *DIY Anti-Aging Cypress Essential Oil Serum*

Ingredients:

- 10 drops of cypress essential oil

- 10 drops of geranium essential oil

- 7 drops of frankincense essential oil

- 1 teaspoon of fresh Aloe Vera gel

- 2 tablespoons of rosehip seed essential oil

- 2 tablespoons of sweet almond oil

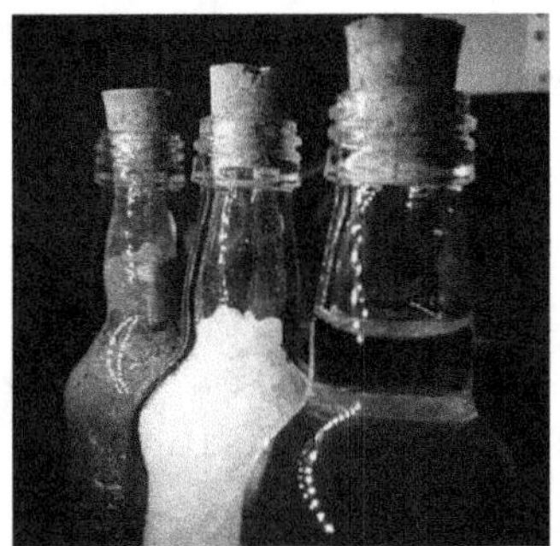

Directions:

Mix your ingredients in a glass bottle. A 2 ounce glass bottle would be good for this recipe. You can use this serum when you get up and just before you go to bed. You only need a small amount of it to cover your face and neck. Don't use too much.

13. DIY Lavender, Peppermint & Frankincense Essential Oil

Ingredients:

- 10 drops of frankincense essential oil

- 10 drops of lavender essential oil

- 5 drops of peppermint essential oil

- 1 tablespoon of beeswax

- 1 tablespoon of Shea butter

- 1/4 cup of extra virgin olive oil

- 3 tablespoons of coconut oil

Directions:

Place the Shea butter, coconut oil, olive oil and beeswax into the top of a double broiler. Heat these ingredients until your beeswax has melted, stirring during this time. Remove from heat and add in your essential oils blending your mixture well. Allow it to cool. Using an electric mixer mix for two minutes. Place your mix in a container of your choice. Apply when you desire to your body and face. Avoid contact with eyes.

14. *Removing Impurities with DIY Essential Oil Facial Mask*

Ingredients:

- 1 drop of peppermint essential oil

- 1 drop of eucalyptus essential oil

- 1 & 1/2 ounces of chamomile tea

- 3 teaspoons of Aloe Vera

- 2 tablespoons of Bentonite, clay

- 3 capsules of activated charcoal

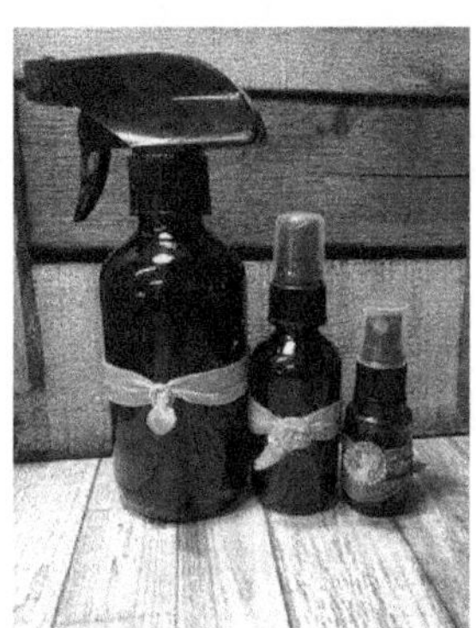

Directions:

This facial mask does as the name suggests and removes impurities from your skin. You apply the mask and leave on for 15 minutes and rinse well. This particular mask works wonders with oily skin and acne. Brew the chamomile tea and melt the Shea butter in a double broiler. After the tea is brewed and the Shea butter is melted mix them together. Mix your Bentonite clay and activated charcoal together in a bowl. Add this mix to the tea mix and stir. Add in your essential oils and Aloe Vera and mix well. Store in an airtight container.

15. DIY Lemon Essential Oil Skin Toner

Ingredients:

- 2 drops of lemon essential oil

- 1/2 tablespoon of fresh lemon juice

- 1 & 1/2 cups of distilled water

Directions:

Add all of your ingredients to a spray bottle and shake well before use. Store in refrigerator and use as needed.

16. DIY Foaming Essential Oil Wash

Ingredients:

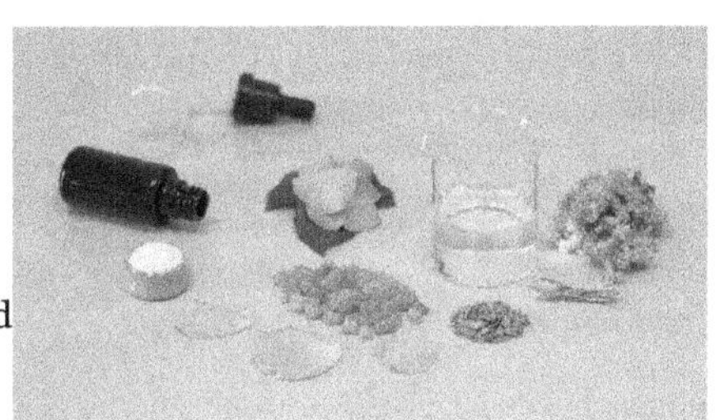

- 10 drops of Ylang-Ylang essential oil

- 6 drops of patchouli essential oil

- 4 drops of lemongrass essential oil

- 1/2 teaspoon of olive oil or sweet almond oil, as carrier oil

- 1/3 cup of Castile soap

- 2/3 cup of distilled water

Directions:

Pour your olive or almond oil along with Castile soap into a container used to dispense foaming soap. Add in your essential oils, swirl the container to fully mix your ingredients. Fill the rest of the container with water. Screw the top on. Use this everyday and you will have radiant glowing skin in no time!

17. DIY Essential Oil Hand Cream

Ingredients:

- 30 drops of your favorite essential oil

- 1/4 cup of Shea butter

- 1/8 of a cup of sweet almond oil

- 1 tablespoon of beeswax

Directions:

Melt the beeswax, sweet almond oil and Shea butter in a double broiler. Once melted remove from heat and add in essential oils. Stir the mix well and pour into jars. You can adjust the amount of beeswax you want to use to make the lotion softer or firmer.

18. DIY Essential Oil Soap Recipe

Ingredients:

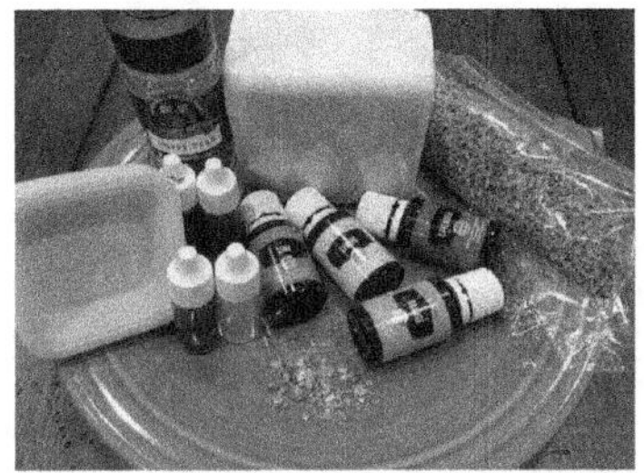

- 5 drops of peppermint essential oil

- 5 drops of tea tree essential oil

- 1 ounce of Castile soap

- 3 ounces of distilled water

Directions:

Mix your ingredients in a glass dispenser. Use it like you would any other liquid soap.

19. *DIY Essential Oil Scalp Stimulation Serum*

Ingredients:

- 5 drops of rosemary essential oil

- 5 drops of chamomile essential oil

- 5 drops of lavender essential oil

- 1 ounce of distilled water

- 1/3 ounce of vodka or alcohol

Directions:

Mix all of the ingredients into a glass jar. You can massage it into your scalp anytime you prefer.

20. *DIY Luminous Essential Oil Face Serum*

Ingredients:

- 4 drops of lemon essential oil

- 4 drops of basil essential oil

- 1 ounce of BDS simple salve

- 4 drops of lavender essential oil

- 4 drops of frankincense essential oil

- 4 drops of geranium essential oil

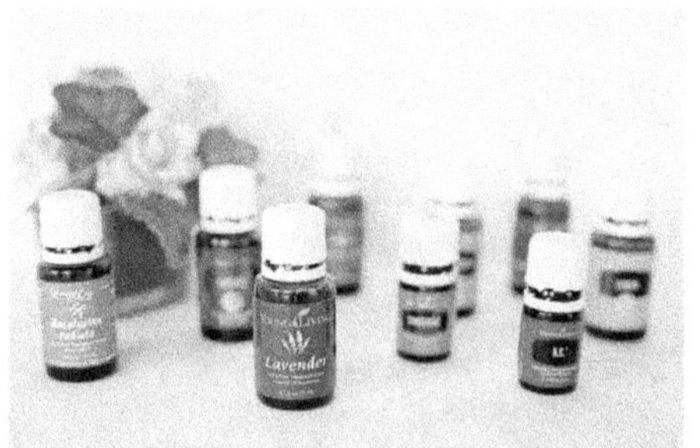

Directions:

Almost fill a one ounce jar with Simple salve, leaving enough room to add your oil. Stir in you essential oils and mix well. Allow the salve to become solid before you cap it.

21. DIY Nutrient-filled Essential Oil Body Lotion

Ingredients:

- 30 drops of rose essential oil
- 20 drops of grapefruit essential oil
- 2 tablespoons of avocado oil
- 4 tablespoons of vegetable oil
- 2 tablespoons of Macadamia oil

Directions:

Mix all of your ingredients in a four ounce bottle. Shake well before each use. This is a wonderful lotion to use after a shower. The oils in it will help to seal in the moisture. You will notice that your skin will become radiant after regular use.

22. DIY Rejuvenating Essential Oil Skin Recipe

Ingredients:

- 6 drops of frankincense essential oil

- 6 drops of lavender essential oil

- 6 drops of patchouli essential oil

- 2 drops of verbena essential oil

- 10 drops of Tamanu carrier oil

- 4 tablespoons of sweet almond oil, use as a carrier oil

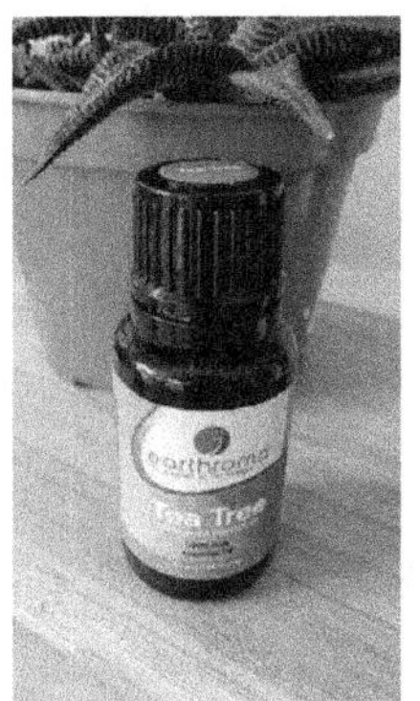

Directions:

In a dark two ounce bottle mix your carrier oil and essential oils and shake well before each use.

23. DIY Lavender Essential Oil Cream for Hands

Ingredients:

- 2 ounces of beeswax

- 3/4 cup of sweet almond essential oil

- 1/4 cup of organic avocado oil

- 1 ounce of vitamin E oil

- 10 drops of lavender essential oil

- 1 cup of warm distilled water

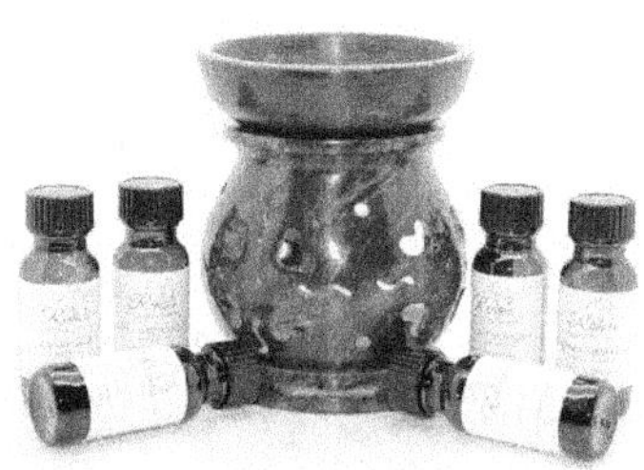

Directions:

Combine the avocado oil, almond oil and beeswax in a double broiler. Heat until the beeswax has melted. Remove from heat, add in the vitamin E oil. Put warm water into a blender. Blend on low as you slowly add in the hot wax and oil. Add in the essential oils and blend until it has creamy texture and thickens. Spoon the cream into jars and secure lids. Allow the cream to cool before you screw on the lids. Store jars in a cool dark place or in the fridge.

24. DIY Essential Oil Moisturizer

Ingredients:

- 1/4 cup of coconut oil

- 12 drops of lavender essential oil

- 12 drops of Melrose essential oil

- 8 drops of Ylang-Ylang essential oil

Directions:

Add your coconut oil into a small glass container or a mason jar will also work. Add in your essential oils and mix well. Use a bit of this mix when you get up in the morning on your face and neck and again before you go to bed. Only use a small amount about the size of 1/2 a pea.

25. DIY Essential Oil Body Butter for Skin Enhancement

Ingredients:

- 2 ounces of Shea butter

- 2 ounces of evening primrose oil

- 10 drops of jasmine essential oil

- 10 drops of frankincense essential oil

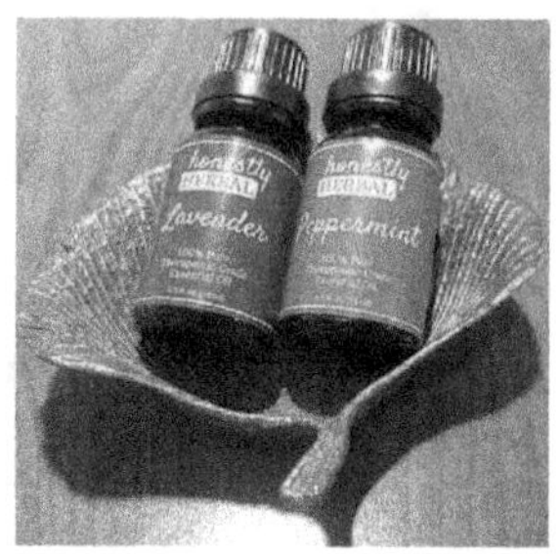

Directions:

In a double broiler melt your Shea butter, but do not get it too hot. Remove from heat and add in your primrose oil and mix. Place the mixture in a bowl to cool in the fridge. Allow it to cool but not yet solid. Remove the mix from fridge and whip using a hand mixer. Add your essential oils into the cream. Mix on low speed until it is blended well. Pour this mixture into glass containers with lids. When this mix sets it will have the texture of butter. You can use it for DIY skin care cream anywhere on your body you want to improve the texture of skin. Do not use this cream on broken skin. It can be used on stretch marks and it smells wonderful and feels so good!

26. DIY Essential Oil Cream for Eczema

Ingredients:

- 25 drops of Melrose essential oil

- 15 drops of lavender essential oil

- 1/4 cup of coconut oil

- 1/4 cup of Shea butter

- 1/2 teaspoon of vitamin E oil

Directions:

Combine the coconut oil and vitamin E oil in a mixing bowl. Add in your essential oils and mix well. Transfer the cream into a container and store at room temperature. If the cream becomes runny store it in the fridge.

27. DIY Essential Oil Body Spray

Ingredients:

- 1 drop of eucalyptus essential oil

- 2 drops of geranium essential oil

- 3 drops of peppermint essential oil

- 4 ounces of distilled water

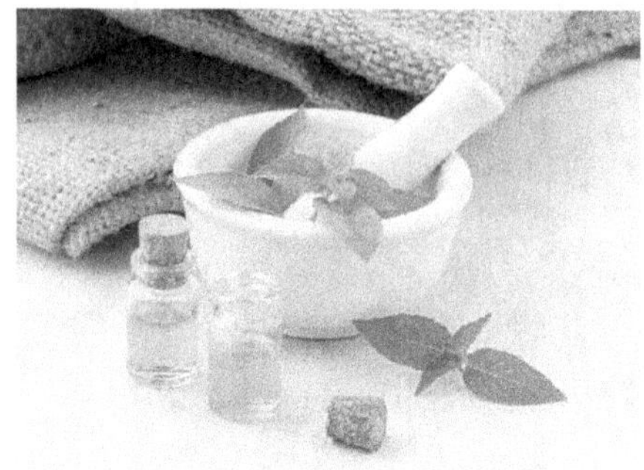

Directions:

Fill a small spray bottle with four ounces of distilled water. Add in your essential oils into the water. Shake the bottle to help to combine the oils and water. Always shake well before each use. You can use this mix on your skin and hair.

28. *Essential Oil Formula for Dark Circles & Brow Lines*

Ingredients:

- 10 drops of frankincense essential oil

- 20 drops of lavender essential oil

- 15 drops of chamomile essential oil

- 2 tablespoons of sweet almond oil

- 2 teaspoons of rosehip oil

Directions:

Drip your chamomile, frankincense, and lavender essential oils into a bottle using a dropper. Add in the rosehip and almond oils at a ratio of 50/50 until you have filled the bottle. Shake well before each use. Apply several drops under your eyes and on your brow before you go to bed.

29. DIY Rosehip Oil for Firming & Toning

Ingredients:

- 10 drops of Cypress or geranium essential oil

- 7 drops of frankincense essential oil

- 2 tablespoons of rosehip oil

- 2 tablespoons of sweet almond oil

Directions:

Mix your ingredients in a small vial or airtight bottle. Choose to use a dark glass bottle to keep out excess light. Apply a few drops of this mix in the morning and in the evening before bed. Sweep drops of mix across your face. You will begin to notice a great improvement on the appearance of your skin.

Conclusion

I hope that you and your loved ones will enjoy the results that you will receive from using my collection of easy to prepare essential oil based skin treatments. You are going to feel so good in just knowing that you are using natural skin treatments on your skin that you made with your own two hands. When you make your own DIY skin care products you know exactly what is being added to them, you no longer have to worry about harmful additives and chemicals being in them. Your skin will show you thanks for the healthy change in skincare products by glowing and looking more healthy than it has in a long time! Not only are you going to replenish your skin but you will also replenish your pocket book with the money you will save on not spending a small fortune on commercial skin products! I wish you and your skin a glowing future—to help ensure that this comes true you are off to a good start in using these DIY essential oil recipes!

I would like to thank you once again for supporting by work, it is much appreciated. I would love to read a review of my book by you on Amazon. Enjoy using this healthy collection of skin care DIY essential oil based recipes! I hope they will give you as much pleasure in their results as they have given me!

FREE Bonus Reminder

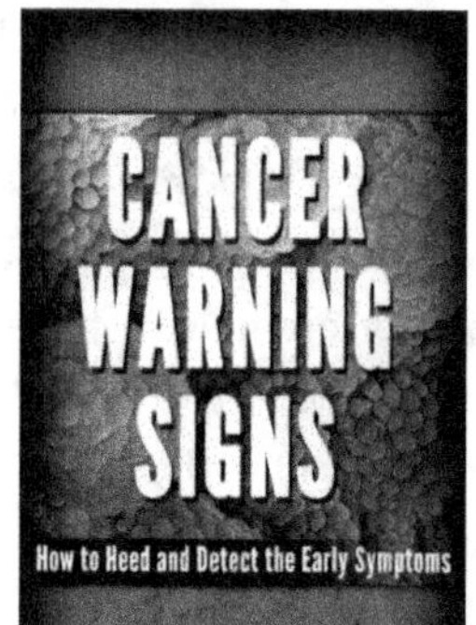

If you have not grabbed it yet, please go ahead and download your special bonus report *"Cancer Warning Signs. How To Heed & Detect The Early Symptoms!"* Simply Click the Button Below

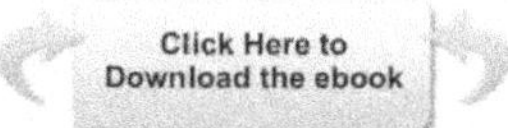

OR **Go to This Page**
http://healthylivingpeople.com/free/

BONUS #2: More Free & Discounted Books or Products
Do you want to receive more Free/Discounted Books or Products?

We have a mailing list where we send out our new Books or Products when they go free or with a discount on Amazon. Click on the link below to sign up for Free & Discount Book & Product Promotions.

=> Sign Up for Free & Discount Book & Product Promotions <=

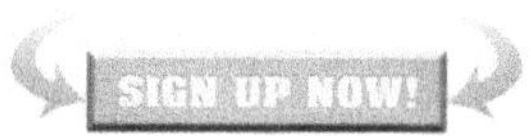

OR Go to this URL
http://zbit.ly/1WBb1Ek